Anissa Zaouak
Houda Hammami
Samy Fenniche

Fixed bullous erythema pigmentosum: a toxidermia not to be ignored

Anissa Zaouak
Houda Hammami
Samy Fenniche

Fixed bullous erythema pigmentosum: a toxidermia not to be ignored

Fixed bullous erythema pigmentosum

Imprint

Any brand names and product names mentioned in this book are subject to trademark, brand or patent protection and are trademarks or registered trademarks of their respective holders. The use of brand names, product names, common names, trade names, product descriptions etc. even without a particular marking in this work is in no way to be construed to mean that such names may be regarded as unrestricted in respect of trademark and brand protection legislation and could thus be used by anyone.

Cover image: www.ingimage.com

This book is a translation from the original published under ISBN 978-620-6-71892-5.

Publisher:
Sciencia Scripts
is a trademark of
Dodo Books Indian Ocean Ltd. and OmniScriptum S.R.L publishing group

120 High Road, East Finchley, London, N2 9ED, United Kingdom
Str. Armeneasca 28/1, office 1, Chisinau MD-2012, Republic of Moldova, Europe
Printed at: see last page
ISBN: 978-620-8-04117-5

BULLOUS FIXED ERYTHEMA PIGMENTOSUM: A TOXIDERMIA THAT SHOULD NOT BE OVERLOOKED DR ANISSA ZAOUAK, PROF HOUDA HAMMAMI, PROF SAMY FENNICHE

TABLE OF CONTENTS

INTRODUCTION

Fixed bullous erythema pigmentosum is a common toxidermia characterised by single or multiple rounded patches that leave a sequelae of pigmented scarring. If the causative drug is reintroduced, the lesions recur at the same site, leaving a residual pigmentation. All ages are affected. The drugs most often responsible are non-steroidal anti-inflammatory drugs, antibiotics and synthetic antimalarials [1,2].EPF is a model of delayed drug hypersensitivity mediated by CD8 T lymphocytes [3]. The onset of this toxidermia is short, ranging from a few days to 2 weeks. The single or multiple cutaneous lesions are of variable cutaneous and/or mucosal topography, most often on the face and trunk.Bullous EPF is a rare clinical form of EPF. It can be localised or generalised.

This rare form is clinically severe and may be confused with other bullous dermatoses such as epidermal toxic necrolysis, erythema multiforme major and autoimmune bullous dermatoses.Few Tunisian studies have focused on this rare and severe form of EPF, hence the interest of this retrospective, monocentric and descriptive study conducted at the Dermatology Department of the Habib Thameur Hospital in Tunis over 17 years (January 2000-December 2016). The aim of this study is to examine the epidemiological, clinical, therapeutic and evolutionary characteristics of erythema pigmentosum bullosa in a hospital series of 16 cases.

METHODS

1. Type of study

This is a retrospective descriptive study of all cases of fixed bullous erythema pigmentosum followed at the Dermatology Department of Habib Thameur Hospital in Tunis over a 17-year period from January 2000 to December 2016.

2. Population of the study

We studied 54 cases classified as erythema pigmentum multiforme. We retained 16 cases of bullous fixed erythema pigmentosa confirmed by anatomopathological examination and a pharmacovigilance investigation.

2.1   Inclusion criteria

We included all cases in which the diagnosis of erythema pigmentosum bullosa was confirmed by anatomopathological study and pharmacovigilance investigation.

2.2   Non inclusion criteria

Records of patients with non-bullous fixed erythema pigmentosum were not included.

2.3 Exclusion criteria

We excluded from this study patients whose medical records could not be used for lack of data.

3 Collection of data

The investigative tool used in the study was a pre-established information sheet containing epidemiological, clinical and paraclinical data, and evolution were recorded. This information was collected from the patients' medical records.

3.1 Epidemiological data

• The patient's age, sex, address, level of education and profession.

• Personal history:

Medical: atopy, drug allergies Surgical

3.2 Data

• History of the disease, onset and duration of symptoms

• Chronology o f onset of skin signs in relation to drug intake

• Consultation period

3.3 Examination data physical

- General signs: general condition, temperature, state of hydration, etc.

- Skin signs: elementary lesions (bullae, macules, erosions, plaques, etc.), the number of lesions and their topography.

- Pleuropulmonary signs: respiratory rhythm, presence of rales, etc.

- Cardiovascular signs: heart rate, blood pressure, etc.

- Signs abdominal :hepatomegaly, splenomegaly, hepatojugular reflux .

3.4 Data from specialist consultations :

- Pharmacovigilance consultation

3.5 Paraclinical data :

Biological tests :

• Blood count (CBC)

• Sedimentation rate (ESR), C reactive protein (CRP), fibrinogen, protein electrophoresis (PEE).

• Transaminases (ASAT/ALAT), Phosphatase alkaline (PAL), Gammaglutamyl-transferase (γGT), Total and direct bilirubin.

• Blood ionogram, creatinine.

3.6 Anatomopathological study :

3.7 Data from the pharmacovigilance survey: imputability score , drug skin tests.

3.8 Diagnostic arguments :

• Positive diagnosis based on clinical criteria and histological confirmation.

3.9 Therapeutic data :

• Local treatments: soothing creams, dermocorticoids

• Systemic treatments: systemic corticosteroids

3.10 Evolution :

Length of follow-up after diagnosis. Evolution: recurrence, recovery, loss of sight.

4. Computer hardware and statistical analysis :

The data for our study were entered using Excel 2010 and analysed using SPSS 20.

5. Bibliographical research :

We used the search engines Pub Med and Google Scholar and the websites Sciencedirect, clinicalkey and Embase.The keywords used were: fixed drug eruption, bullous fixed drug eruption, drug eruption

6. Ethical considerations and conflict of interest :

We have no conflicts of interest to declare.

1. Epidemiology :

1.1 Impact :

The impact of erythema pigmented pigment is estimated

0.9/10000consultants/year.

1.2 Age :

In our study, the mean age was 42.85 years, with extremes ranging from 2 and

a half to 80 years.

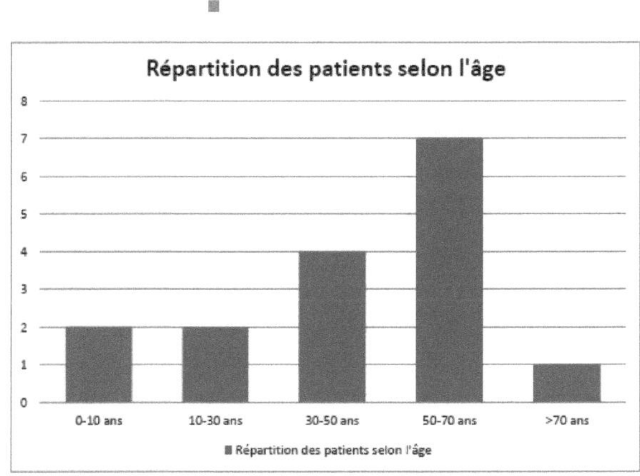

Figure 1: Age distribution of patients

1.3 Gender :

In our study, the M/F sex ratio was 1.28.

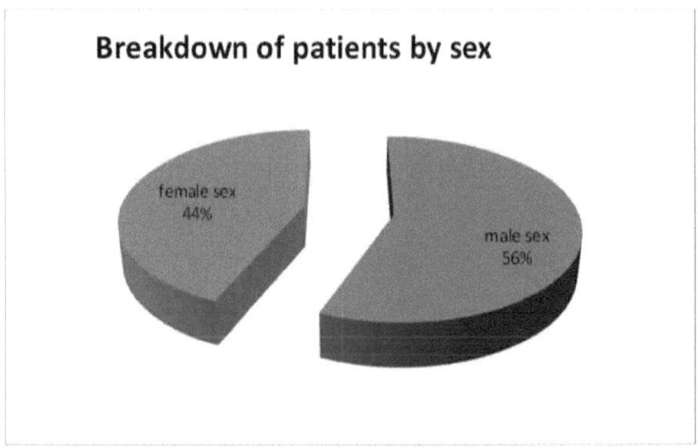

Figure 2: Breakdown of patients by gender

1.4   Breakdown of patients by age and gender :

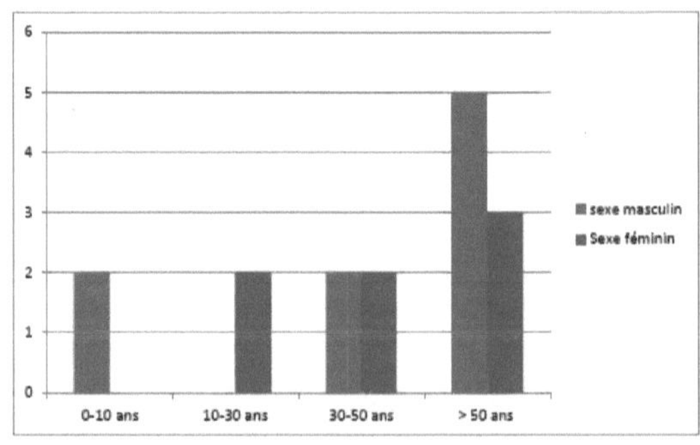

Figure 3: Breakdown of patients by age and sex

2. Clinical study :

2.1 Clinical aspect of bullous EPF :

In our patients, the clinical presentation was dominated by the presence of tense bullae with haemorrhagic content resting on erythematopurple skin. In some patients, the bullae had ruptured, leaving extensive post-bullous erosions over purplish skin. Skin involvement was localised in 8 patients and generalised in 8 patients. Isolated cutaneous involvement occurred in 7 patients, isolated mucosal involvement in 3 patients and mucocutaneous involvement in 6 patients.

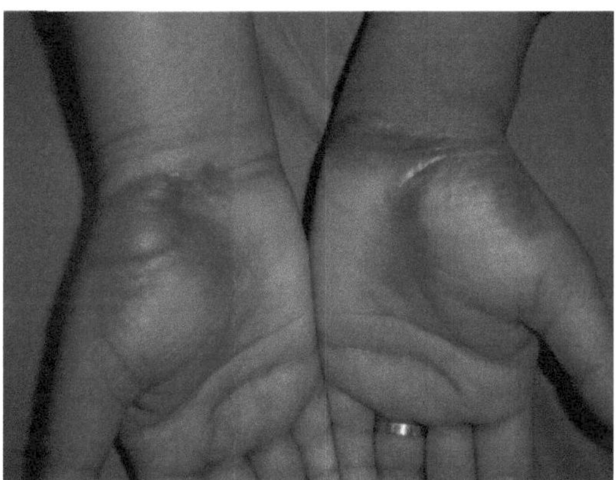

Figure 4: Purplish patches on the palms of the hands surmounted by tense bullae with haemorrhagic content (case 11).

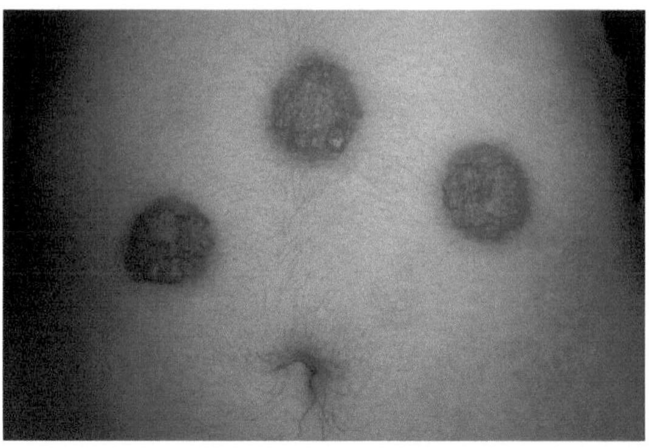

Figure 5: Three purplish patches surmounted by vesiculo-bubbles on the abdomen (case 16)

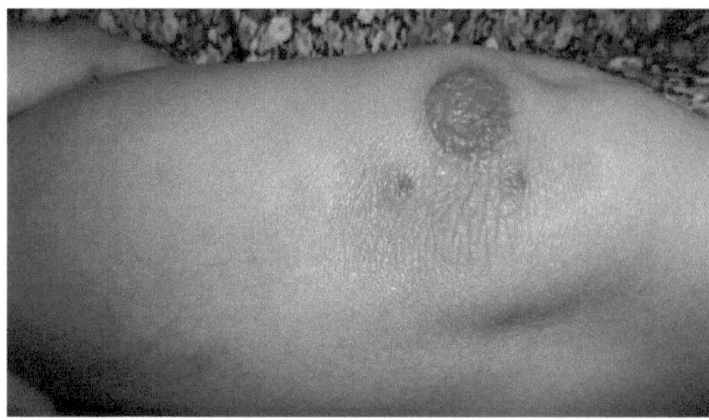

Figure 6: Bullae in the elbow with haemorrhagic content (case 9)

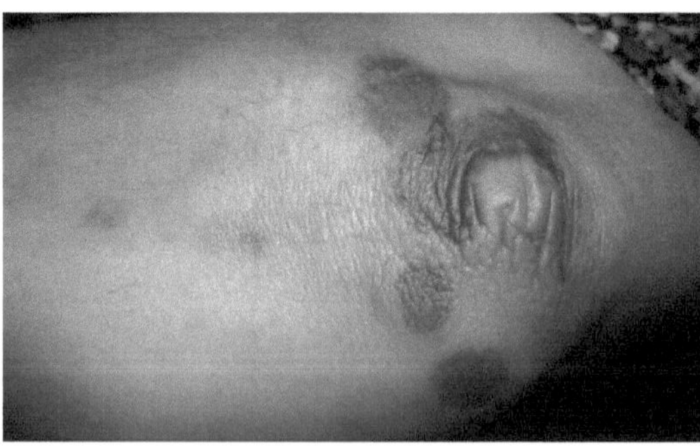

Figure 7: Post-bullous erosions on the elbow (case 9)

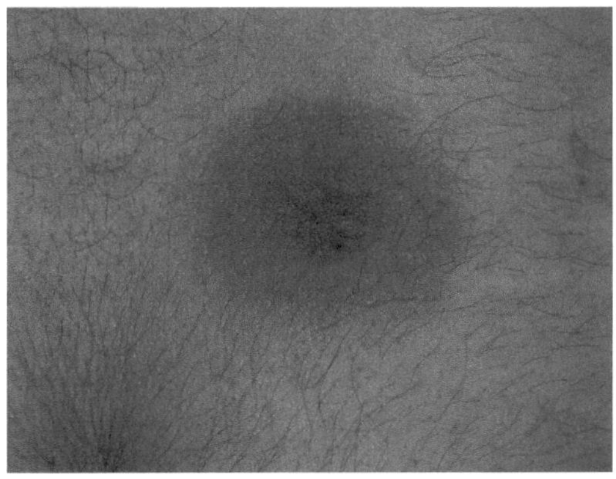

Figure 8: Rounded erythematoviolaceous plaque with bullous centre (case 2)

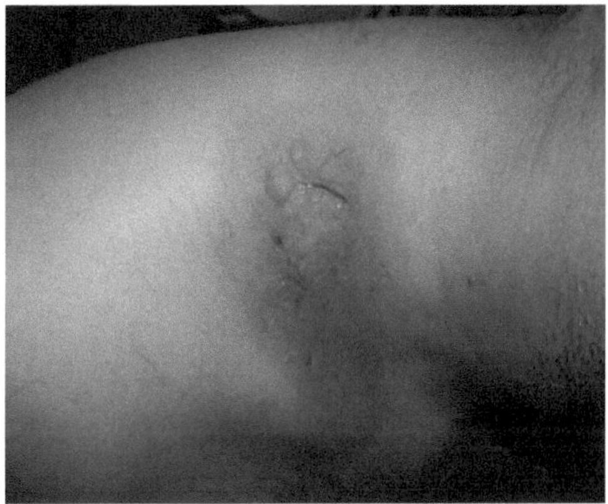

Figure 9: Post-bullous erosion of the shoulder on an erythema-violet background (case 6)

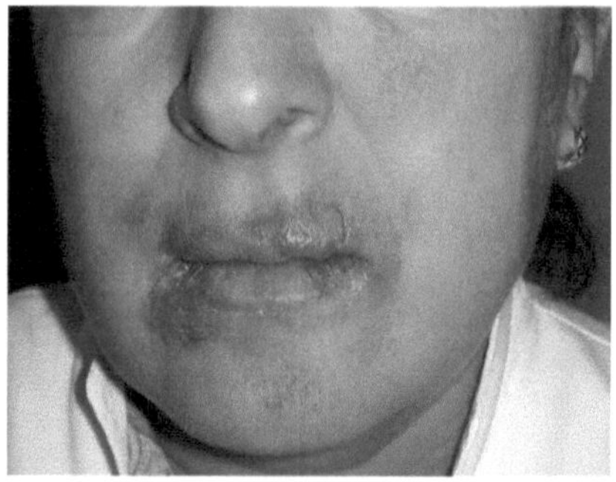

Figure 10: Multiple erythema-violaceous patches on the face, with bullae in places (case 14)

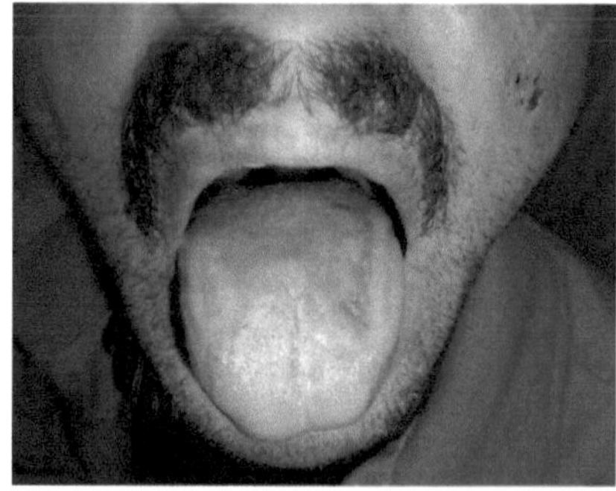

Figure 11: Linear erosion at the tongue (case 7)

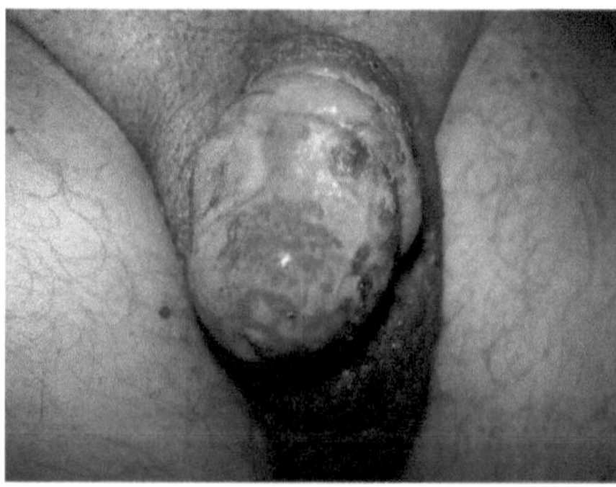

Figure 12: Post-bullous erosive plaque of the glans penis and balanopreputial fold (case 6)

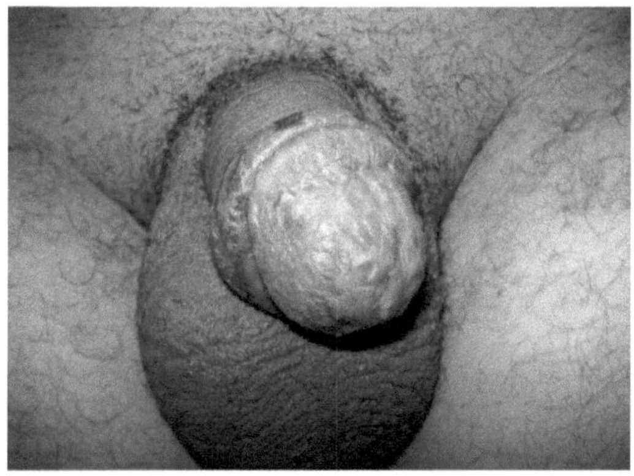

Figure 13: Scab-covered erosions of the glans penis and balanopreputial

fold (case 8)

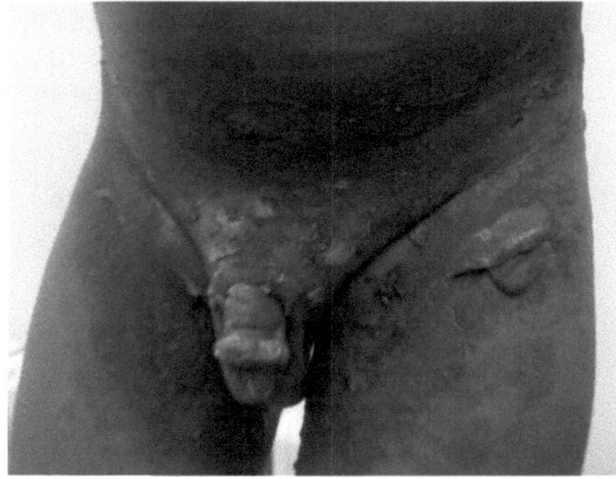

Figure 14: Vast placard of bullae and post-bullous erosions of the perineum

in a child (case 1)

2.2 Number of lesions :

In our series, the number of bullous lesions varied from one plaque with a bullous centre or one post-bullous erosion to several bullae and post-bullous erosions.

2.3 Location of lesions :

In our series, cutaneous involvement was isolated in 7 cases, isolated mucosal involvement of the buccal or genital mucosa in 3 cases and cutaneous-mucosal involvement in 6 cases.

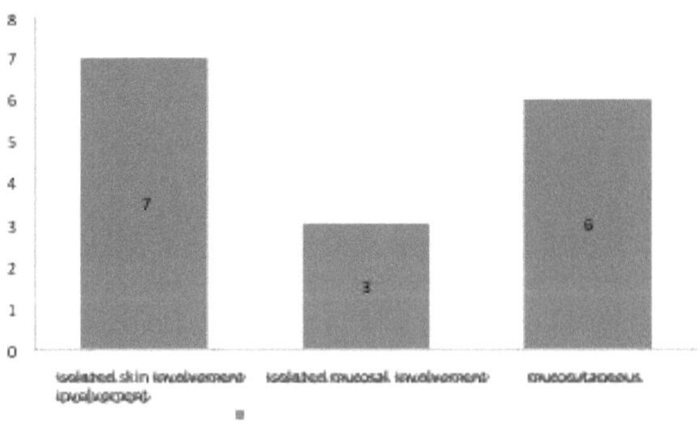

Figure 15: Distribution of skin involvement by site

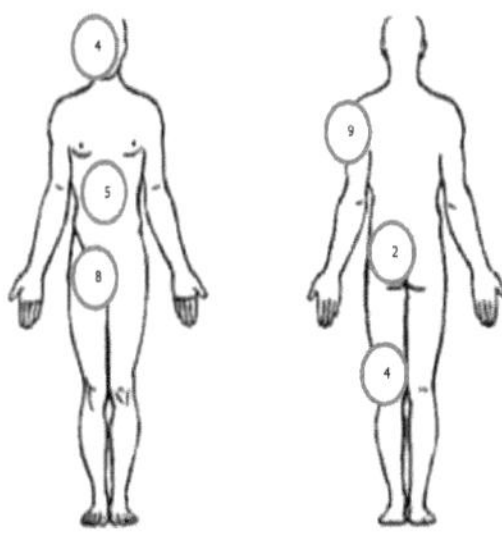

Figure 16: Location of bullous EPF lesions

3. Chronology of appearance of lesions by in relation à the drug intake:

The onset of skin lesions varied from a few hours to a few days.

4. Drugs implicated in the genesis of EPF :

The main drugs implicated in the genesis of erythema pigmentosum bullosa were NSAIDs in 12 cases, followed by antibiotics in 4 cases.

Table I: Drugs implicated in fixed bullous erythema pigmentosum

Offending drug	Number of cases
Non-steroidal anti-inflammatory drugs	12 cases
Mefenamic acid (Inflamyl®)	4 cases
Diclofenac (Voltarene®)	1 case
Ibuprophen (Ibuprophen®)	4 cases
Sodium tenoate (Toufilex®)	2 cases
Oxicam (Roxan®)	1 case
Antibiotics	4 cases
Doxycycline (Doxycycline®)	2 cases
Sulfamethoxazole (Bactrim®)	2 cases

5. Anatomopathological study :

Anatomopathology revealed keratinocytic necrosis, sometimes confluent, which may be responsible for epidermal detachment. The mononuclear infiltrate affected the superficial and deep dermis and consisted of lymphocytes, neutrophils and eosinophils of interstitial and perivascular topography. Sometimes there was an accumulation of melanophages in the superficial dermis. Direct immunofluorescence tests in 4 cases were negative.

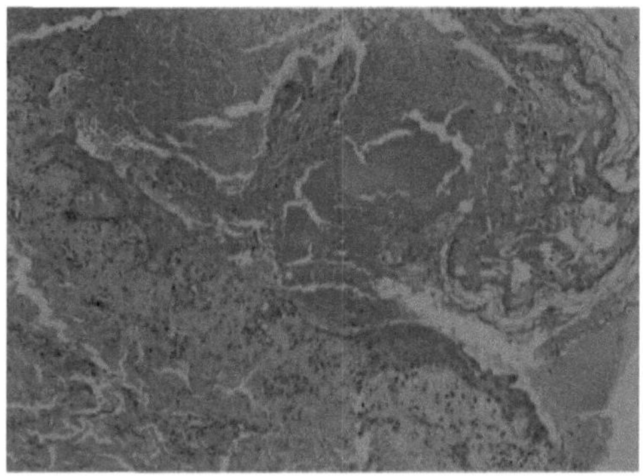

Figure 17: Detached epidermis in necrotic subepidermis topped by

laminated keratin (HEX40)

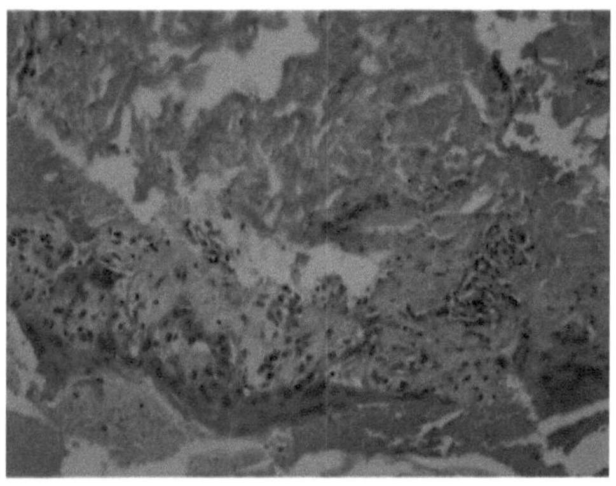

Figure 18: Inflammatory infiltrate of the dermis made up of lymphocytes,

PNN and PNE (HEX100)

6. Treatment :

This table summarises the treatments taken by our patients in our series.

<h2 align="center">Table II: Treatments received by patients</h2>

Treatment received	Number of patients
General corticosteroid therapy and dermocorticoids	8 patients
Dermocorticoids	8 patients
Soothing creams	3 patients

7. Evolution :

All our patients progressed well with local and/or general treatment. Patients who underwent a pharmacovigilance investigation had no recurrence.

8. Summary table :

<h2 align="center">Table III: Summary table of all observations</h2>

Patient	Age	Gender	Episode of	Time to onset of	Head quarters	fr o m	Medicines	Score	Score
			the bubbly EPF	the eruption	EPF bullous		incriminated	imputab ility	of imputabili tee (Begaud (Naranjos hold) et al)
1	2 years and half	M	1er episode	24 Heures	located		NSAIDS	7	I3
2	42 years old	M	1er episode	24 Heures	located		ATB (Bactrim)	7	I3
3	55 years old	M	Recurrence	A few hours	located		NSAIDS	8	I4
4	61 years	M	Recurrence	Not specified	Located		NSAIDS	7	I3

	old							
5	80 years old	M	1er episode	A few days	widespread	NSAIDS	7	I3
6	51 years old	M	Recurrence	24 Heures	widespread	ATB (Doxy)	8	I4
7	42 years old	M	Recurrence	8 Hours	widespread	NSAIDS	9	I4
8	41 years old	M	1er episode	3 days	widespread	ATB (Bactrim)	7	I3
9	60 years old	F	1er episode	2 days	widespread	NSAIDS	7	I3
10	50 years old	F	Recurrence	A few days	located	NSAIDS	8	I4
11	50 years old	F	1er episode	24 Heures	Located	ATB (Doxy)	7	I3
12	52 years old	F	1er episode	A few days	widespread	NSAIDS	7	I3
13	8 years old	M	1er episode	24 Heures	located	NSAIDS	8	I3
14	56 years old	F	Recurrence	A few days	widespread	NSAIDS	8	I4
15	26 years old	F	Recurrence	24 Heures	widespread	NSAIDS	8	I4
16	19 years old	F	1er episode	3 days	located	NSAIDS	7	I3

DISCUSSION

1. Reviews of our study :

Our study reported the main clinical features of fixed bullous erythema pigmentosum, a rare toxidermia. It can affect both men and women, adults and children. In our series, the drugs incriminated in the genesis of erythema pigmentosum bullosa were mainly NSAIDs and antibiotics. Because of its bullous nature, this toxidermia can simulate several bullous dermatoses such as pemphigus, bullous pemphigoid, erythema multiforme, but also toxidermia with a severe prognosis such as toxic epidermal necrolysis, hence the interest of this study. In our series, mucosal involvement was frequent, making diagnosis sometimes difficult due to the absence of residual pigmentation. The limitations of our study are essentially the small number of patients (16), explained by the rarity of this type of bullous toxidermia.

2. Epidemiology :

2.1 Impact :

The incidence of EPF varies from one country to another, ranging from 2.5% to 22%. The incidence of the bullous variant has not been specified in the literature due to the diagnostic difficulties of this variant [4].

2.1.1. Worldwide :

Table IV: Main series on erythema pigmentum multiforme worldwide

Author	Year	series	Country	Durationnof the study
Nnoruka et al[5]	2006	81	Nigeria	3 years
Brahimi et al [6]	2010	59	France	3 years
Atadokpédé and al[7]	2011	155	Benin	11 years old
Ognongo-Ibiaho and al[8]	2012	54	Congo	27 months
Saka et al[9]	2012	321	Togo	6 years old
Rahman et al[10]	2013	120	Bangladesh	Not specified
Jung et al[11]	2014	134	Korée	11 years old
Heng et al[12]	2014	126	Singapore	5 years
Kavoussi et al [13]	2015	30	Iran	10 years

2.1.2. In Tunisia :

In our series,the incidence a was estimatedà 0.9/10000 patients/year, indicating the rarity of this toxidermia.

In Tunisia, 3 main studies were carried out on erythema pigmentum fixans, as detailed in Table V.

Table V: Main studies on erythema pigmentum fixans in Tunisia

Author	Year	series	Duration study	Tunisia	Work
Zaiem[14]	2010	21 cases	4 years	Tunis	Memory
Kastalli[15]	1999	120	12 years old	Tunis	Thesis
Aouina[16]	2016	221cas	15 years old	Tunis	Thesis
Our study	2017	16 cases	17 years old	Tunis	Memory

2.2 Age :

Bullous EPF can affect all ages, with a predominance of young adults. The mean age in our series was 42.85 years. In our series, we had two children with bullous EPF. Bullous erythema pigmentosa affects people of all ages, including children and the elderly [4,17].

2.3 Gender :

In our series, the M/F sex ratio was 1.28. Bullous EPF can affect men and women equally without gender predominance [18].

3. Pathophysiology of fixed erythema pigmentosa :

Erythema pigmentum fixans is a model of delayed hypersensitivity mediated by CD8+ T lymphocytes. Intraepidermal CD8 lymphocytes play a major role in the development of the disease. In lesions of erythema pigmentum fixata, these T lymphocytes have a memory effector phenotype. These CD8 lymphocytes are detected in lesions of fixed erythema pigmentosa and are responsible for tissue damage [3].

4. Clinical study :

4.1 Clinical aspect :

Erythema pigmentosum bullosa can be localised or generalised. In our series, bullous EPF was localised in 8 patients and generalised in 8 patients. Generalised EPF is characterised by numerous (>10) well-defined vesiculobullous oedematous plaques on erythematous, purplish skin involving at least 3 sites. In our series, 8 patients had genital involvement, which is common in bullous EPF, mainly affecting the glans penis in male patients. Mucosal bullous fixed erythema pigmentosum can have a bullous, erosive, aphthoid or erythematous appearance [1,2].

4.2 Headquarters :

In our series, the most frequent location was the upper limbs (9 patients), followed by the external genitalia (8 patients) and then the lower limbs (6 patients). This has been confirmed in various series in the literature.

5. Drugs responsible for bullous EPF :

In our series, the drugs incriminated in the genesis of erythema pigmentosum bullosa were essentially NSAIDs and antibiotics. Table VI summarises the different drugs implicated in the genesis of EPF bullosa in the literature.

Table VI: Drugs responsible for erythema pigmentosum bullosa in the literature

Medicines	Author	Year
Doxycycline	Nitya et al [19] Podder et al [20]	2013 2016
Tadalafil	Grimaux et al [21]	2016
Bromhexine	Vide et al [22]	2016
Fluconazole	Slawinska et al [23]	2017
Azithromycin	Das et al [24]	2016
Paracetamol	Agarwala et al [25]	2016
Product fromcontrast iodized	Epskamp et al [26]	2016
Phenytoin	Jain et al [27]	2015
Pseudoephedrine	Bellini et al [28]	2016
Ciprofloxacin	Nair et al [29]	2015
Vaccine from the fever yellow	Sako et al [30]	2014
Influenza vaccine	Garcia Doval et al [31]	2001
Flurbiprofen	Balta et al [32]	2014
Metronidazole ovule	Hermida et al [33]	2011
Naproxen	Bandino et al [34]	2009
etoricoxib	Duarte et al [35]	2010
flecainide	Knapp et al [36]	2009
Nimesulide	Kumaran et al [37]	2004
Rifampicin	Goel et al [38]	2001
Paclitaxel	Young et al [39]	1996
Metronidazole per os	Bhargava et al [40]	1996
Erythromycin	Naïk et al [41]	1976

6. Anatomopathological study :

Pathological examination revealed interface dermatitis with lymphocytes at the dermal-epidermal junction and basal vacuolation of epidermal cells associated with keratinocyte necrosis. PNNs, PNEs and intraepidermal granulocytic abscesses are found within the dermal infiltrate. Melanophages may be found in the superficial dermis. The histological differential diagnosis may be erythema multiforme or bullous pemphigoid [2].

7. Diagnosis: Positive diagnosis :

The diagnosis is suspected clinically and confirmed histologically. For the drug in question, a good anamnesis and the pharmacovigilance investigation are used. Intrinsic (Appendix 4) and extrinsic drug imputability scores are available, which can help to determine drug imputability, especially in polymediated patients [42]. The definitive diagnosis of drug imputability is the drug skin patch test or the oral provocation test.

7.1 Differential diagnosis :

The main differential diagnosis of generalised bullous erythema pigmentosum is toxic epidermal necrolysis. The table below summarises the differences between generalised bullous EPF and toxic epidermal necrolysis.

- If genital form: diagnosis may be made with a herpetic recurrence or pemphigus

- If bullous form: in addition to toxic epidermal necrolysis, the diagnosis can be made with erythema multiforme or dermatoses. autoimmune bullous diseases such as pemphigus or linear Ig A dermatosis [43,44].

Table VII: Differential diagnosis of fixed bullous erythema pigmentosa

	Generalized bullous EPF	Necrolysis toxic epidermal
Age	>60 years	30-60 years old
History of taking medication or history of an episode similar	frequent	rare
Time between the drug intake and the eruption	Short <2 days up to 14 days	14 days +or - 7 days
Normal skin	Wide intervals	Few intervals
Bullous lesions	Well limited Involvement palmar-plantar Pigmentation sub secondary	Confluent, symmetrical Atypical targets
Re-epidermisation	Early <10 days	Long >15 days
Healing	No pigmentation, pigmentation underlying	Yes,scars mucous membranes
Surface skin epidermal detachment	Moderate	High
Mucosal damage	Limited Few erosions <=1 site	Involvement mucous membrane major >=2 sites
General condition	Retained Temperature<38.5° C	General state of health Temperature >=38.5° C
Histology	Infiltration significant of P E cells and	Necrosis epidermal extensive

	dermal melanophages Low levels of intraepidermal CD56 and cells expressing granulysine	High levels of CD56 and granulysin + intraepidermal
Levels serum of granulysine	Low	High

8. Treatment :

8.1 Therapeutic means :

Treatment is essentially symptomatic.Aetiological treatment is essentially based on stopping the suspected treatment while the cause is confirmed by an appropriate pharmacovigilance investigation.

- Antiseptic baths

- Topical creams: dermocorticoids and healing creams

- Mouthwash and eye drops

- Analgesics

- Nursing care: application of non-adhesive dressings to post-bulbar erosions

- Oral corticosteroid therapy at a dose of 0.5mg/kg/d, cyclosporine, IGIVs

8.2 Indications :

- If localized form not too extensive: treatment with dermocorticoids and healing creams

- If generalised bullous form with systemic signs: hospitalisation in an intensive care unit, systemic corticosteroid therapy, cyclosporine or IGIV depending on the severity of the clinical picture [45,46].

- If the ocular mucosa is affected: instillation of antibiotic and anti-inflammatory eye drops

- If the oral mucosa is affected: mouthwash with chlorhexidine

9. Evolution and prognosis :

Bullous fixed erythema pigmentosum usually has a good prognosis, with rapid re-epidermisation and lower mortality [44,47].

10. Skin tests and fixed erythema pigmentosum :

Patch testing in erythema pigmentum fixans is a practical diagnostic method for determining the drug responsible. Drug patch tests should be performed on the site previously affected by EPF, especially if several molecules are involved [48,49].According to the recommendations of the European Society of Contact

Dermatitis, patch tests can be carried out with the drug in its marketed form diluted 30% in petroleum jelly.

11. Treatment of fixed bullous erythema pigmentosum :

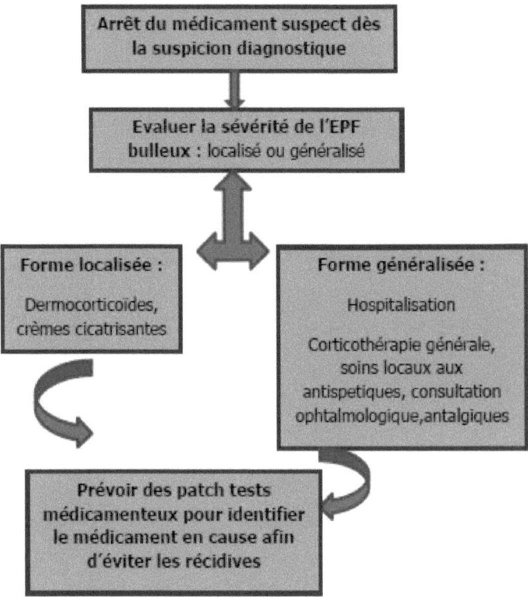

Figure 19: Treatment of fixed bullous erythema pigmentosa

CONCLUSIONS

Bullous fixed erythema pigmentosum is a common toxidermia characterised by single or multiple rounded patches that leave a pigmented sequellar scar. If the causative drug is reintroduced, the lesions recur at the same site, leaving a residual pigmentation. All ages are affected. The drugs most often responsible are non-steroidal anti-inflammatory drugs, antibiotics and synthetic antimalarials [1,2]. EPF is a model of delayed drug hypersensitivity mediated by CD8 T lymphocytes [3].Bullous EPF is a rare and severe clinical form of EPF. It can be localised or generalised. This rare form is clinically severe and may be confused with other bullous dermatoses such as epidermal toxic necrolysis, erythema multiforme major and autoimmune bullous dermatoses.The aim of our study was to investigate the epidemiological, clinical, therapeutic and evolutionary characteristics of erythema pigmentosum bullosa in a hospital series of 16 cases. We conducted a retrospective, monocentric, descriptive study at the Dermatology Department of the Habib Thameur Hospital in Tunis over 17 years (January 2000-December 2016), including 16 cases.In our series, the incidence of fixed erythema pigmentosa was evaluated at 0.9 cases. /10,000 consultants/year, indicating the rarity of this toxidermia. The average age was 42.85 years. Bullous EPF can affect all ages, with a predominance in young adults. Children may also be affected (2 cases in our series). The sex ratio M/F was 1.28. EPF affects both men and women, with no gender predominance.In our patients, the clinical presentation was dominated by the presence of tense bullae with haemorrhagic content on erythematous skin. purplish. In some patients, the bullae ruptured, leaving vast post-bullous erosions on purplish skin. Skin involvement was localised in 8 patients and generalised in 8 patients. Isolated cutaneous involvement occurred in 7 patients, isolated mucosal involvement in 3 patients and mucocutaneous involvement in 6 patients. The most frequent site of lesions was the upper limbs, followed by the external genitalia and then the lower limbs, which is consistent with the data in the literature.The onset of skin lesions varied, ranging from a few hours to a few days after taking the drug.The main drugs implicated in the development of erythema pigmentosum bullosa were NSAIDs in 12 cases, followed by antibiotics in 4 cases.Anatomopathological studies carried out on all patients revealed keratinocytic necrosis, sometimes confluent, which may be responsible for epidermal detachment. The mononuclear infiltrate involved the superficial and deep dermis and consisted of lymphocytes, neutrophils and eosinophils of interstitial and perivascular topography.The episode of bullous EPF was inaugural in 9 patients and a recurrence in 7 patients. A pharmacovigilance investigation was carried out in all patients to identify the drug involved, and the intrinsic drug imputability score ranged from probable I3 in 10 patients to very probable I4 in 6 patients. Two patients had skin patch tests identifying the suspect drug. Eight patients were treated with systemic corticosteroids and 8 patients were treated with local corticosteroids and the suspect drug was discontinued, with a good clinical outcome. The strengths of our study lie in the fact that we have attempted to identify this rare bullous variety of EPF, which may be confused with other autoimmune bullous dermatoses or other more severe toxidermias such as toxic epidermal necrolysis. The aim of this study was to describe the clinical features of this toxidermia, which frequently affects mucous membranes, and to highlight the contribution of pharmacovigilance investigations in identifying the suspect drug and thus preventing future recurrences.

REFERENCES

1. Valeyrie-Allanore L, Lebrun-Vignes B, Bensaid B, Sassolas B, Barbaub A. Fixed pigmented erythema: Epidemiology, physiopathology, clinical features, differential diagnosis and therapeutic management. Ann Dermatol Venereol. 2015;142(11):701-6.

2. Ozkaya E. Fixed drug eruption: state of the art. J Dtsch Dermatol Ges. 2008;6(3):181-8.

3. Shiohara T, MizukawaY. Fixed drug eruption: a disease mediated by self-inflicted responses of intraepidermal T cells. Eur J Dermatol. 2007;17:201-8.

4. Lee AY. Fixed drug eruptions Incidence, recognition and avoidance. Am J Clin Dermatol. 2000;1(5):277-85.

5. Nnoruka EN, Ikeh VO, Mbah AU. Fixed drug eruption in Nigeria. Int J Dermatol. 2006;45(9):1062-5

6. Brahimi N, Routier E, Raison-Peyron N, Tronquoy AF, Pouget-Jasson C, Amarger S et al. A three-year-analysis of fixed drug eruptions in hospital settings in France. Eur J Dermatol. 2010;20(4):461-4.

7. Atadokpédé AF, Adégbidi H, Yédomon HG, Koudoukpo C, Agbessi N, Gnossike J et al. Fixed drug eruption in Cotonou, Benin from 1998 to 2008. Ann Dermatol Venereol. 2011;138(4):320-2.

8. Ognongo-IbiahoAN,AtandaHL. Epidemiological study of fixed drug eruption

in Pointe-Noire. Int J Dermatol. 2012;51(1):33-5.

9. Saka B, Kombaté K, Médougou BH, Akakpo S, Mouhari-Toure A, Boukari T et al. Fixed drug eruption in dermatology setting in Lomé (Togo): a retrospective study of 321 cases. Bull Soc Pathol Exot. 2012;105(5):384-7.

10. RahmanMH.Fixed drug eruption in Bangladeshi population: confirmed by provocative test. Int J Dermatol. 2014;53(2):255-8.

11. Jung JW, Cho SH, Kim KH, Min KU, Kang HR. Clinical features of fixed drug eruption at a tertiary hospital in Korea. Allergy Asthma Immunol Res. 2014;6(5):415-20.

12. Heng YK, Yew YW, Lim DS, Lim YL. An update of fixed drug eruptions in Singapore.J Eur Acad Dermatol Venereol. 2015;29(8):1539-44.

13. Kavoussi H, Rezaei M, Derakhshandeh K, Moradi A, Ebrahimi A, RashidianHet al. Clinical Features and Drug Characteristics of Patients with Generalized Fixed Drug Eruption in the West of Iran (2005-2014). Dermatol Res Pract. 2015;2015:236703.

14. Zaïem A. Apport des patch tests dan le diagnostic de l'érythème pigmenté fixe [Mémoire]. Medicine: Tunis; 2010. 47p

15. Kastalli S. Erythema pigmentum fixata: clinical diagnosis and drug liability [Thesis]. Medicine: Tunis; 1999. 76p

16. Aouina H. Clinical diagnosis and drug imputability of erythema pigmentum fixans [Thesis]. Medicine: Tunis; 2016. 73p

17. Raman M, Pandhi RK. Fixed drug eruption in infancy. Indian Pediatr. 1993;30(1):110-1.

18. Sharma VK, Dhar S. Clinical pattern of cutaneous drug eruption among children and adolescents in north India. Pediatr Dermatol. 1995;12(2):178-83.

19. Nitya S, Deepa K, Mangaiarkkarasi A, Karthikeyan K. Doxycycline induced generalized bullous fixed drug eruption-A case report. J Young Pharm. 2013;5(4):195-6.

20. Podder I, Chandra S, Das A, Gharami RC.Doxycycline Induced Generalized Bullous Fixed Drug Eruption. Indian J Dermatol. 2016;61(1):128.

21. Grimaux X, Bigot P, Leclec'h C. Bullous fixed drug eruption of the glands due to tadalafil: A case report. Prog Urol. 2016;26(8):435-6.

22. Vide J, Moreira C, Cunha AP, Baldaia H, Magina S, AzevedoF. Generalized bullous Fixed Drug Eruption due to Bromhexine. Dermatol Online J. 2016;15:22(7).

23. Sławińska M, Barańska-Rybak W, Wilkowska A, Nowicki R. Bullous fixed drug eruption due to fluconazole, mimicking herpes simplex.Clin Exp Dermatol. 2017;17:22-7.

24. Das A ,Sancheti K , Podder I , Das NK. Azithromycin induced bullous fixed drug eruption.

Indian J Pharmacol. 2016;48(1):83-5.

25. Agarwala MK, Mukhopadhyay S , Sekhar MR, Peter CD. Bullous Fixed

Drug Eruption Probably Induced by Paracetamol.Indian J Dermatol. 2016;61(1):121.

26. Epskamp C, Snels DG, Yo GL, Zuetenhorst HJ, Hamberg P. Bullous fixed drug eruption in a patient with metastatic renal cell carcinoma induced by iodinated contrast during pazopanib treatment. Eur J Dermatol. 2016;26(2):207-8.

27. Jain A, Gupta N. Multifocal Bullous Fixed Drug Erruption Due To Phenytoin: A Lesson Learned!J Clin Diagn Res. 2015;9(12):OD04-5.

28. Bellini V, Bianchi L, Hansel K, Finocchi R, Stingeni L. Bullous nonpigmenting multifocal fixed drug eruption due to pseudoephedrine in a combination drug: clinical and diagnostic observations. J Allergy Clin Immunol Pract. 2016;4(3):542-4.

29. Nair PA. Ciprofloxacin induced bullous fixed drug reaction: three case reports. J Family Med Prim Care. 2015;4(2):269-72.

30. Sako EY, Rubin A, Young LC. Localized bullous fixed drug eruption following yellow fever vaccine.J Am Acad Dermatol. 2014;70(5):e113-4.

31. García-Doval I, Rosón E, Feal C, De la Torre C, Rodríguez T, Cruces MJ. Generalized bullous fixed drug eruption after influenza vaccination, simulating bullous pemphigoid. Acta Derm Venereol. 2001;81(6):450-1.

32. Balta I, Simsek H, Simsek GG. Flurbiprofen-induced generalized bullous fixed drug eruption. Hum Exp Toxicol. 2014;33(1):106-8.

33. Hermida MD, Consalvo L, Lapadula MM, Della Giovanna P, Cabrera HN. Bullous fixed drug eruption induced by intravaginal metronidazole ovules, with positive topical provocation test findings. Arch Dermatol. 2011;147(2):250-1.

34. Bandino JP, Wohltmann WE, Bray DW, Hoover AZ. Naproxen-induced generalized bullous fixed drug eruption. Dermatol Online J. 2009;15(11):4.

35. Duarte AF, Correia O, Azevedo R, do CarmoPalmares M, Delgado L. Bullous fixed drug eruption to etoricoxib--further evidence of intraepidermal CD8+ T cell involvement. Eur J Dermatol. 2010;20(2):236-8.

36. Knapp CF 3rd, Cooke ER, Sheehan DJ. Bullous fixed drug eruption caused by flecainide. J Am Acad Dermatol. 2009;60(2):e3.

37. Kumaran S, Sandhu K, Saikia UN, Handa S. Nimesulide induced bullous fixed drug eruption of the labial mucosa. Indian J Dermatol Venereol Leprol. 2004;70(1):44-5.

38. Goel A, Balachandran C. Bullous necrotizing fixed drug eruption with hepatitis due to rifampicin. Indian J Lepr. 2001;73(2):159-62.

39. Young PC, Montemarano AD, Lee N, Sau P, Weiss RB, James WD. Hypersensitivity to paclitaxel manifested as a bullous fixed drug eruption. J Am AcadDermatol. 1996;34:313-4.

40. Bhargava P , Mathur DK, Agarwal US, Bhargava R . Severe bullous fixed drug eruption due to metronidazole mimicking a localized form of toxic epidermal necrolysis. Indian J Dermatol Venereol Leprol. 1996;62(1):55-6.

41. Naik RP, Singh G. Bullous fixed drug eruption presumably due to

erythromycin. Dermatologica. 1976;152(3):177-80.

42. Bégaud B, Evreux JC, Jouglard J, Lagier G. Imputability of unexpected or toxic effects of drugs. Thérapie. 1985;40:111-8.

43. Bataille M, Vonarx M, Vermersch-Langlin A. Illustration of diagnostic and prognostic difficulties during the early stages of generalized bullous fixed drug eruptions. Eur J Dermatol. 2017;27(1):86-88.

44. Özkaya E. Oral mucosal fixed drug eruption: characteristics and differential diagnosis. J Am Acad Dermatol. 2013;69(2):e51-8.

45. Mockenhaupt M. Severe drug-induced skin reactions: clinical pattern, diagnostics and therapy.J Dtsch Dermatol Ges. 2009;7(2):142-60.

46. Malviya N , Cyrus N , Vandergriff T , Mauskar M . Generalized bullous fixed drug eruption treated with cyclosporine. Dermatol Online J. 2017;15:23(2).

47. Lipowicz S, Sekula P, Ingen-Housz-Oro S, Liss Y, Sassolas B, Dunant A et al. Prognosis of generalized bullous fixed drug eruption: comparison with Stevens-Johnson syndrome and toxic epidermal necrolysis. Br J Dermatol. 2013;168(4):726-32.

48. Zaïem A, Charfi O, Sahnoun R, Lakhoua G, Daghfous R, Aïdli S et al. The contribution of epicutaneous tests in erythema pigmentum fixans. Rev Fr Allergol. 2014;54(3):258.

49. Andrade P, Brinca A, Gonçalo M. Patch testing in fixed drug eruptions- a

20-year review. Contact Dermatitis. 2011;65(4):195-201.

50. Naranjo CA, Busto U, Sellers EM, Sandor P, Ruiz I, Roberts EA, et al. A method for estimating the probability of adverse drug reactions. Clin Pharmacol Ther. 1981;30(2):239-45.

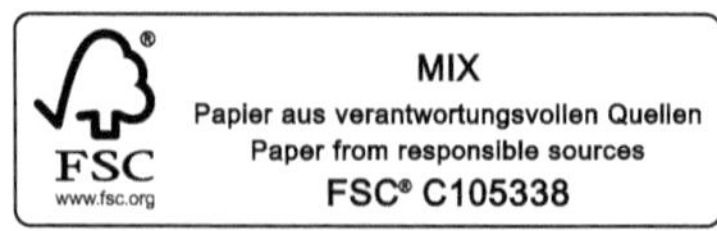

Printed by Books on Demand GmbH, Norderstedt / Germany